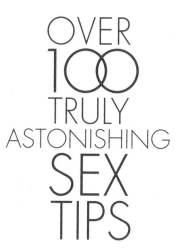

OVER
100
TRULY
ASTONISHING
SEX
TIPS

THIS IS A CARLTON BOOK

Text and design copyright © 2000 Carlton Books Limited

This edition published by
Carlton Books Limited 2000
20 Mortimer Street
London W1N 7RD

A CIP catalogue for this book is available
from the British Library.
ISBN 1 85868 910 4

Editorial Manager: Venetia Penfold
Art Director: Penny Stock
Design: DW Design
Production: Alexia Turner and Garry Lewis

Printed in Italy

OVER 100 TRULY ASTONISHING SEX TIPS

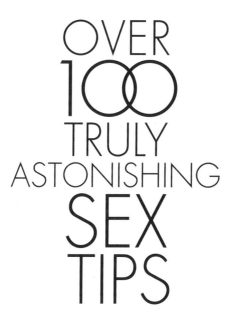

LISA SUSSMAN

CARLTON
BOOKS

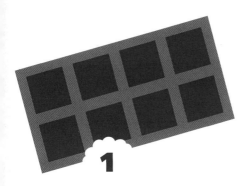

1

Eating chocolate can also hike up your PEA count. Try smearing chocolate body-paint (available from sex shops) or chocolate syrup over each other's bodies, and then lick it off. Yum!

2

Scatter **rosebuds** over your bodies and the bed before you make love. The petals will become crushed between your sweaty bodies, gorgeously scenting your sex. Who said life wasn't a bed of roses?

Ask him to give you a **belly orgasm**. Sit erect on the edge of a chair. Your lover should stand behind you and place his hands, pointing downwards, in a triangle on your abdomen – and rub. You'll feel your ovaries get warm and tingle a bit. Breathe deeply. You'll soon begin to feel a sexy buzz.

Get some **sleep**. One study from an American sleep centre found that women who reported going to bed later than usual 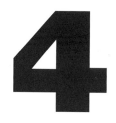 one night were rarely in the mood for making love the next. A possible reason for this is that when you're getting enough shut-eye, your levels of the stress hormone, cortisol, drop. Fatigue gives this hormone a chance to build up, which may erode sexual appetite.

Get him to tickle your **Ahh! zone**. Known as the anterior fornix zone, it's a soft, squashy bump located on the front wall of the vagina, between the G-spot and the cervix. This hot spot has awesome bliss potential – studies show that stroking here helps women to become easily lubricated and experience single or multiple orgasms during sex

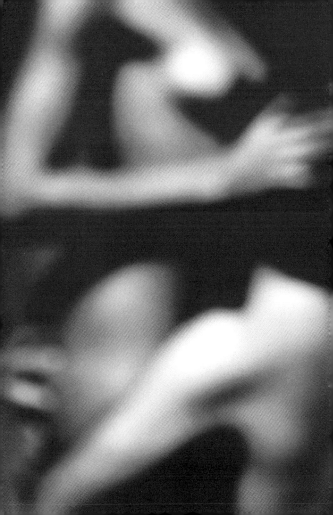

6 Wash each other's **hair**. Besides being incredibly sensual (think how good it feels at the hairdresser's), the Kinsey Institute New Report on Sex found that good grooming was even more important to lovers than penis or breast size!

Ears are an underrated erogenous zone. The lobe and the small area behind the shell have a hot line to the nerves. Stimulation from a darting tongue or a light, probing finger can be a powerful aphrodisiac – especially when combined with heavy breathing into the ear. Scientists call the phenomenon the auriculogenital reflex, and trace its origins to a nerve in the ear canal. Some men find it so exciting they actually climax from it.

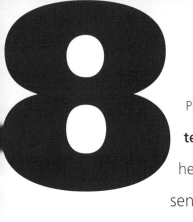

Playing with **temperature** heightens the sensations because your blood vessels will alternately expand and contract. Run an ice-cube over each other's **hot** skin, or spray your sheets with ice-**cold** water.

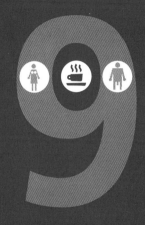

Heat things up even more. Take a cup of hot fruity tea to bed with you, sip it and then wrap your mouth around your lover's most sensitive parts. Ask him to do the same. You'll melt with pleasure.

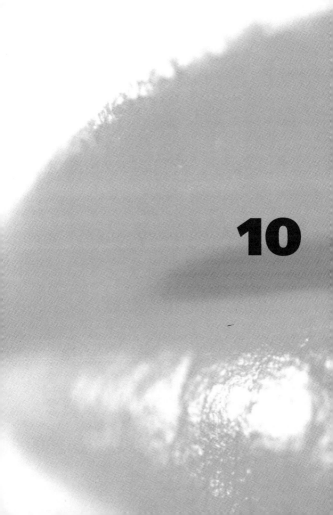

10

Say 'Ooommmm'. In one study, meditation breathing and relaxation exercises significantly raised levels of dehydroepiandrosterone (DHEA), the hormone that revs up our sex drive.

Masturbate. It's a delicious cycle. The more frequent a woman's sexual activity – alone or with a partner – the better her sex life. Research has found that women who pleasure themselves regularly have increased sexual desire, more orgasms, greater sexual and relationship satisfaction and higher self-esteem. Makes you want to give yourself a hand!

Prime your body for a hot and heavy love session. Power squats will build up the muscles that are exercised during sex, giving you added stamina for the main event **(your orgasm)**. Stand up, feet slightly further than shoulder-width apart, arms straight out in front of you for balance. Push your hips and bum back, and bend your knees forward (no further than your toes). Then straighten your legs. Do three sets of 15 reps, three times a week.

13

Tickle the roof of his mouth with your **tongue**.

14

Give
his
sacrum a
stroke (and
get him to return
the favour). This
small dent, located just
above the crease of the
bum, (aka the Bermuda
Triangle of love) is extremely
responsive when massaged in a
circular motion with your thumb.

Come – er – prepared. Red-hot lovemaking is a sure thing if you keep your libido on a low boil throughout the day by fantasizing about body-bonding with your lover later on. One study by the Center for Sexual Health at Tulane Medical Center in New Orleans, found that when women have a mental rehearsal for sex, especially if they have a history of orgasm no-shows, their bodies become more sexually responsive within **30 seconds**, once the action really gets going.

16

Resist the urge to make love for a few days, and then set an exact date and time to break the fast. In the meantime, tease each other mercilessly with deep kissing, erotic massage, and light stroking, especially on your favourite hot spots. Sometimes, building anticipation is the most glorious foreplay of all.

17

Learn how to tell a farmer's-daughter joke. Research by the Society for the Scientific Study of Sex found that women who see the **funny side of life**, and are amused by sex-related jokes, are lustier and have higher levels of sexual satisfaction than their more serious sisters.

Call in late to work. The prime time for him to have sex is 9 am. This is when his testosterone level peaks, so physiologically it's all systems go. (You'll probably feel more in the mood, too, as a woman's testosterone cycles often echo her partner's.)

18

With more than **72,000 nerve endings**, your hands are very receptive sex tools. Make the most of every single nerve ending by putting on blindfolds and caressing each other from head to toe, lightly tickling with your fingertips, kneading with your fingers, pressing with your palms, circling with your whole hand and patting gently with the sides of your hands.

Make things **sizzle** by coating his testicles in minty toothpaste before intercourse. The ever-increasing heat sensation this produces will make you both squirm with pleasure. Afterwards, you can lick off any residue (although it won't help to prevent cavities!).

20

21

Give him **a kiss** he'll feel all the way down to his toes. Lie facing each other and press your lips together tenderly *à la* Clark Gable and Vivien Leigh in *Gone with the Wind*. While you can keep the connection for as long as you want, Tantric teachers recommend you hold it for at least seven seconds, in order to experience an all-over glow.

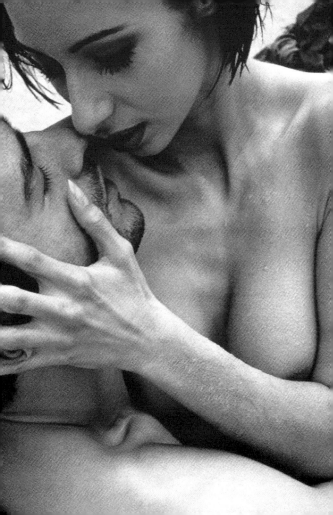

Ignite a secret **hot spot**. Because urine is expelled through the urethra, we don't usually think of this tiny area of tissue just below the clitoris as a sexual point, but Kevin McKenna, PhD, an associate professor of physiology and urology at Northwestern University Medical School, found that it's a possible trigger for orgasm when pressed. It's also a good place to shift your lover's attention, post-orgasm, when your clitoris feels too sensitive for direct stimulation, but you're still in the *mood for pleasure*.

Give each other a body-to-body **rubdown**: ask your man to lie face down on a soft supportive surface like the bed or a thickly carpeted floor. Start crawling on top of his back, rubbing it with the front of your body and hands. Work your way downwards, finishing with your breasts wedged in the crease below his buttocks and your genitals somewhere mid-leg. Your clitoris will sizzle from the pressure of your movements, and the sensation of your breasts on his bottom will tantalize him. If you do this immediately after bathing while your bodies are still moist, it will make things sensually slippery, without losing any of the fabulous friction.

23

24

Even the shade of your boudoir or lingerie can affect your rapture rating. In a study at Loyola University in New Orleans, both sexes thought that the **three most erotic colours** (in descending order) were red-orange, dark blue and violet. And the least erotic? Grey.

S t y l e
your pubic
hair. But instead
of a complete shave
with a razor (which can
leave a decidedly un-sexy
itch), trim each other with
electric clippers. Bonus: the vibration
from the clippers will add a delightful
tingle. If he's not sure he wants a haircut
down there, tell him that the shorter the hair,
the bigger his organ will look.

Touch

for

your

own

pleasure,

not

your

partner's.

Act like a **vampire** and go for the neck. (Do NOT draw blood!) Gently kissing and sucking the points to the immediate left and right of the Adam's apple drives 1,000 volts of pleasure through the spine.

27

Have a two-in-one orgasm. Some sex experts believe we experience two types of orgasmic sensations – the first is a sharp twinge that occurs when the clitoris or base of the penis is stimulated; the second is a warm melting feeling that happens when the inside of the vagina or the shaft of the penis is aroused to climatic heights. Experience both types, one after the other in a single love fest, and you've had what's

2

called a blended orgasm. He caresses your clitoris until it's almost too sensitive to touch; then he moves his attention to the interior of your vagina. Once you are feeling totally aroused, he moves back to your clitoris. Meanwhile, you are doing the same with his penis, moving from the base to the shaft to the head, and back again. Keep on going for an hour of mind-warping climatic bliss.

8

Rub a few drops of **lavender oil** in your hair. According to the Smell and Taste Treatment and Research Foundation in Chicago, this scent turns men into lust-crazed beasts (or near enough). Your olfactory turn-on? Cucumbers (no phallic jokes, please).

29

30

Take your **vitamins and minerals**. According to nutritionists, vitamins B and E and zinc enhance the efficiency of the nervous system, leading to a stronger libido and better orgasms.

Rub his inner **G-spot**. Get him to lie on his back. Sit between his legs and massage the shaft of his penis with one hand, using lots of moisture and a circular stroke. When he's getting close to orgasm, use your other hand to caress his perineum firmly (the hair-free patch of skin at the base of his scrotum). Sit back and watch his toes curl.

Ask your lover to give you a **three-finger** caress. By bringing together the pointer, middle and ring finger of his hand, he will be able to massage every sensitive nerve ending on your clitoris.

32

③②

33

For a more **intense** orgasm, lie on your back with your head lower than the rest of your body, either by lifting your hips with your hands, with the help of some supporting pillows under your hips, or by positioning yourself so that your head hangs slightly off the bed. This increases blood flow to your brain and changes your breathing, both of which can add to arousal.

Try *dok el arz*, which means 'pounding in the spot'. An ancient Arabian position, it manages to give him the deep penetration that he desires, and your clitoris the attention it craves: the man sits down with his legs stretched out, the woman then places herself astride his thighs, crossing her legs behind her man's back. Lining things up, the woman guides her lover into her. She then places her arms around his neck while he embraces her waist and helps her rise and plunge upon him.

34

Light a
candle.
Undress.
Explore
each
other for
as long
as the
candle
burns.
When it
sputters,
go for
your
climax in
the dark.

THIRTY-FIVE

36

Comedy isn't the only thing that requires good timing. Pencil in sex during the four days following **ovulation** (around the third week of your cycle), when your testosterone levels peak. Studies show that women are more likely to masturbate, initiate intercourse and reach orgasm easily during these days (caveat: they are also more likely to get pregnant).

37

Give each other an alternative orgasm by stimulating one of these acupressure hot spots: use the heel of the hand to gradually increase pressure in the centre of the crease where the thigh joins the front of the torso, rub the area between the mid-thigh and the genitals, or use a forefinger and index finger to massage the temples in gentle circular motions.

Spice up foreplay with the **alphabet game**. Take turns making capital letters with your tongue very slowly on each other's genitals. You might make it to 'M'…

38

39 Pump it up. Your heart, that is. Thirty minutes of aerobic exercise three times a week can do wonders for your sex life – and your orgasm power: studies show it boosts testosterone levels (making you more in the mood for sex), tones cardiovascular endurance (enabling you to last longer), increases blood-vessel diameter and blood volume (making vaginal tissue more sensitive), and improves circulation (making orgasms more forceful).

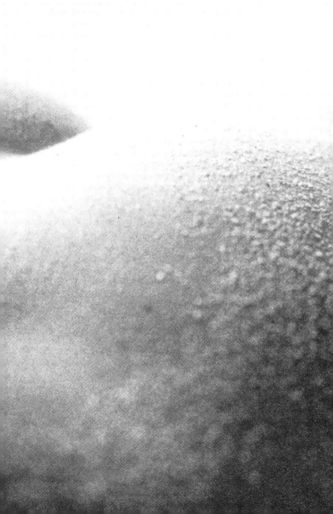

40 Remember to **breathe**. According to a study by the Center for Marital and Sexual Studies in Los Angeles, most women tend to unconsciously hold their breath during sex, which kills arousal. Instead, try taking slow, regular breaths as you feel your excitement build. The more you can control your breaths, the deeper your orgasm will be.

41

Having a sexy dream at night can make you sizzle during the day. With practice, you can induce a **siesta orgasm** by indulging in your favourite turn-on before you start counting sheep at night.

Feed each other an ambrosial fruit salad. According to the Smell and Taste Treatment and Research Foundation in Chicago, oranges increase penile blood flow by 20 per cent, strawberries spur sexual satisfaction, and spices like nutmeg and cinnamon make you want to do it again and again…

42

43

Play some Harry Connick Jr. A study from the National Opinion Research Center in Chicago found that **jazz** listeners had the most sex. The fluidity of the music also makes you move more rhythmically – especially when you're horizontal.

44

The biggest problem with **orgasms** is that his erupt speedily while yours come at a more leisurely pace. But you can keep him to your rhythm with a tender tug. Using your thumb and fingers, encircle his scrotum (not testicles!) as he nears climax. Squeeze firmly and pull down lightly for a few seconds. He'll groan with ecstatic pleasure if you do it right, with pain if you are too rough. So remember to take it easy – practice makes perfect.

Introduce him to your **breasts**. According to a survey in the *Practical Encyclopedia of Sex and Health*, only 50 per cent of women say they enjoy having their breasts fondled during foreplay – mainly because they're in the hands of men who fumble the ball. Tell him what pleases you by putting your hand over his and caressing the area together.

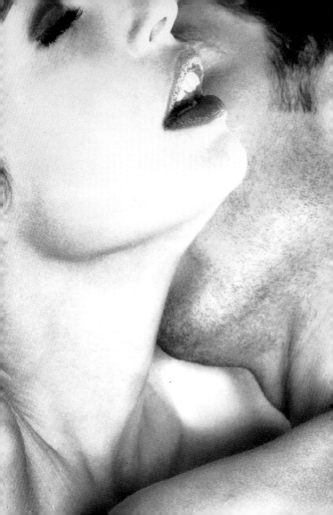

Exchange **tongue baths** – starting from the fingertips, lick each other's bodies all over, leaving not a single patch unwashed.

47

Do one thing differently. If you normally nibble his ear, nibble his nipple. If you always end up on top, do it lying on your sides. An Archives of Sexual Behaviour study showed that making **one small variation** in your standard sex routine can help lovemaking to become thrilling all over again.

If you're almost at orgasm and get stuck, sex researchers Julia Heiman and Joseph LoPiccolo have found that deliberately *tensing* your legs, stomach, arms or feet will send you over the edge.

48

Check *Old Moore's Almanac* for the lunar schedule. A report published in the *New England Journal of Medicine* states that women are 30 per cent more sexually active (read: more likely to rip his clothes off) during a **full moon** than at any other time of the month. 49

50 According to Masters & Johnson, orgasms are really just a sweet release of incredible tension. So boost the intensity of yours by hovering around the 'Ohhh-I'm-almost-there' spot for as long as possible. Get as close to peaking as you can, then relieve the pressure by getting your lover to stimulate a less sensitive area of your body. Repeat until you're **ready to burst**.

Have him lick your **upper lip**. Just about every ancient Eastern sex philosophy claims that this site is the key to a woman's clitoris, and touching it is guaranteed to create

cosmic sparks.

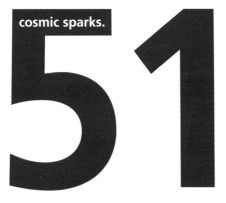

51

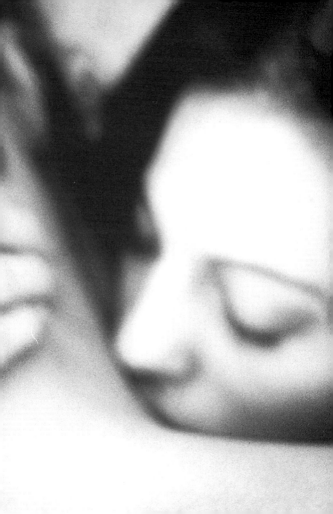

52

Forget oysters. The best aphrodisiac (although, perhaps not the tastiest) is a diet low in lard. The lower your body fat, the higher your levels of testosterone and DHEA. Low blood-cholesterol levels can also reduce plaque build-up in the arteries, increasing circulation and blood flow to the genitals. *Bon appétit*.

Read any **Harold Robbins** book. Rent a sexy video like *Bitter Moon* or *The Lover*. Racy images jump-start your sexual response by raising levels of phenulethulamine (PEA), carnal chemicals that flood your brain when it's buzzed on sex.

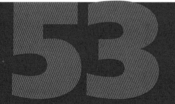

The penis has its own **hot spot** just waiting for the right touch. The raphe is a seam, which you can both see and feel, that runs lengthways along the scrotum. Hit his moan zone by lightly tracing your fingers along the line, moving from his bottom forwards and up towards the base of his penis.

Go straight to **sleep**. Sex in the middle of the night, after you've both clocked up a couple of hours' shut-eye, can be much more profound.

55 ZZZZ z z z

Time your **foreplay**. A Kinsey report found that only 7.7 per cent of women

56 whose lovers spent 21 minutes or longer on pre-penetration fun and games failed to reach orgasm.

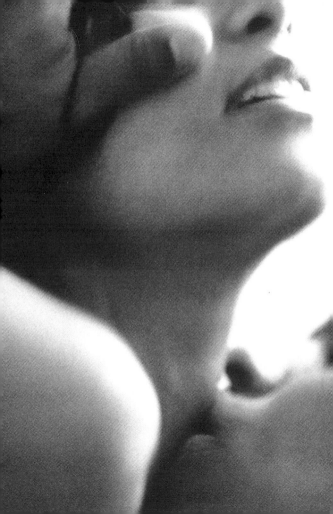

For an indirect pleasure prep, gently press the area about 6.5 cm (2½ inches) below your **belly button** for about three minutes. This helps promote blood flow, which stimulates the entire pelvic area. Oh, and you can expect a mind-blowing orgasm, too.

57

58

Ribbed **condoms** are supposed to add to a woman's pleasure. But turn one inside out and those little ridges can do wonderful things to his penis, too (mix in a dab of water-based lubrication to avoid breakage).

Skip the perfume wrist spritz. In Ayurvedic medicine, the ancient Indian science of health and healing, the lower stomach is considered to be the centre of a woman's **sexual stamina**. Dabbing the area with fragrances that are

59 supposed to have aphrodisiac qualities – such as neroli, jasmine, sandalwood and patchouli – will set the scene for a steamy night. As you become aroused, the increased blood flow to your pelvis generates heat in the area, helping to release the fragrance – and unleash your animal magnetism.

60°

Get hot – literally. Soak in a warm bath, take a steam or Jacuzzi at your gym, sunbathe (slap on the SPF first), jump up and down until you're sweating, make love on sheets fresh from the dryer. According to a Czechoslovakian study, heat depletes our body's store of stress hormones, making us more in the mood for *l'amour*.

61

Climb **on top** when making love. Experts agree that when a woman is in this position, three marvellous things happen: the forward-facing wall of the vagina (the epicentre of all of her genital hot spots) and the clitoris are more easily stimulated; she can control the angle and depth of penetration more easily; and she becomes more involved in the act of intercourse – all of which add up to a more achievable and impressive orgasm.

X

Buy a **porn flick**. Yes, YOU. An Archives of Sexual Behaviour study found that women get just as turned on watching erotica as men do. However, since most of the films available are for the male market, you might want to check out Femme Productions, which produce films specifically for women and couples.

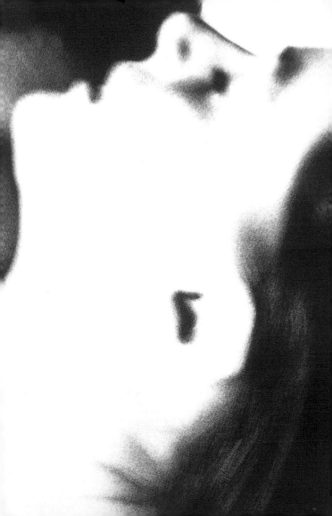

Blow his...mind. Put both of his balls in your mouth at once. Use one hand to circle the top of the sac, and gently pull it down to bring the balls together into a neat swallowable package. Being extremely careful to cover your teeth with your lips, take the sac in your mouth and give him a tongue lashing he'll never forget.

64 Anthropologists call a reddened mouth a **'genital echo'**, a term that includes all body parts with a passing resemblance to a love organ. Drive the point home by applying some bright red lipstick and giving him a blow job (making sure he has a good view).

Equip yourselves with torches and **turn off the lights**. Take turns turning the high beam on each other. Whatever part of the body is lit up has to be caressed for five minutes with the lightee's mouth or hand.

65

Sex in the bath can actually dry out your juices. If you're not using latex birth control, add a few drops of oil to the water to keep things lubricated.

67

More **thrusting** does not necessarily mean more fun. The most sensitive nerve endings in the vagina are actually near the opening, so shallow penetration is really better for you. Since this also allows constant stimulation to the head of the penis and, specifically, the hypersensitive frenulum, both of which are squeezed by the vaginal muscles located near the vaginal opening, you won't hear any complaining from him, either.

During **foreplay**, pull back your hair so that

he can see your face.

Try something new **three times**. The first time, you may be worrying about bending your knees, elbows or both at the proper angle; the second time, you will be thinking about how to make it work for you, but the third time you try you'll probably find that you're able to relax and go with the flow.

Give each other a deep **tonsil-touching** kiss, every time you meet. Experts agree that smooching can be more intimate than sex (which may be why prostitutes often draw the line at kissing). When psychotherapist Sylvia Babbin, PhD, investigated the number of times an average couple kissed, she counted only four-and-a-half pecks per day – including hello, goodbye, good morning and good night.

70

71

Deep-throating is a learned technique. To swallow his penis as fully as possible during oral sex, throw your head back as far as it will go. This opens up the throat and allows you to accept an elongated object without causing your gag reflex to react. Lying on your back with your head over the edge of the bed and breathing through your nose is the most comfortable way to maintain this position.

72 Make him stand to attention. A study at a recent American urology conference established that taking 80 mg of Ginkgo biloba a day can boost his potency (and your pleasure). Seems the herb increases blood flow by relaxing the arteries. But don't expect overnight results – it can take several weeks before you notice a difference.

Move in together. A national survey of Family and Households found that men and women who live together have the most sex, making love more often than non-cohabiting couples, even after they marry.

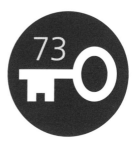

74

Make intercourse **clitoral-friendly**. Research shows that only about 30 per cent of women have regular orgasms from penetration. But when they use something called the coital alignment technique, the odds improve to 77 per cent. Begin with your man on top in the missionary position. He should then slide slightly forward, causing his pelvis to override yours. Instead of thrusting (and completely bypassing the clitoris), you rock your pelvis up while he responds with a downward pressure, so the penis shaft stimulates the clitoris directly, and possibly the G-spot, too.

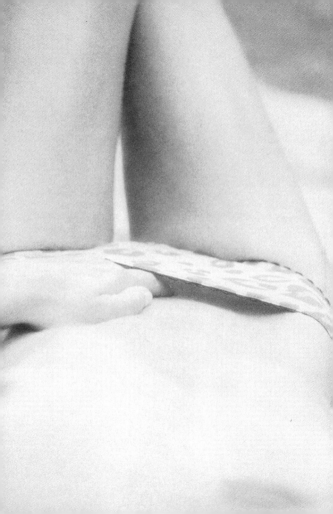

75

According to the Kinsey Institute, the average

man thinks about sex at least once every

half-hour. Use this knowledge!

Ride a **ROLLER COASTER**

– or anything else that makes you quake with fear. According to research conducted by psychologist Judy Kuriansky, PhD, **76** for Universal Studios Amusement Park in Florida, experiences that make our stomachs flip over result in a surge of adrenaline and endorphins, which can make us feel more lusty.

77

Reorganize your bedroom for a more amorous atmosphere. According to **feng shui**, the ancient Chinese art of creating a harmonious living environment, if your bed has a view of the whole room, with nothing blocking the door, your lovemaking will buzz with energy and understanding.

Telling a man you **want** him is the sexiest thing you can do. It packs the same erotic punch as informing him that his team's won, he's won the Lottery AND you've bought him a Harley Davidson. You don't have to be obvious. Simply turn a hello peck into a mini make-out session, and he'll soon get the picture.

78

GO TO THE PUB. According to research cited in *Nature* magazine, one to two glasses of alcohol elevates testosterone levels in women – especially women who are ovulating or on the Pill. But get him to stick to water – booze has the opposite effect on male testosterone LEVELS.

Emptying your bladder makes it easier to stimulate your **G-spot**.

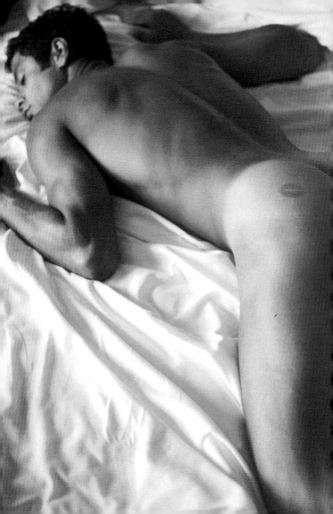

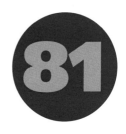

81

Here's a good argument for investing in a **nicotine patch**: a new study reveals that quitters have more orgasms than when they smoked. Tobacco chemicals supposedly constrict blood flow to the vagina and penis, and may lower testosterone levels.

Unlike women, men don't have built-in **lubricants**. Give your hand a lick before caressing his penis to help make things deliciously squishy.

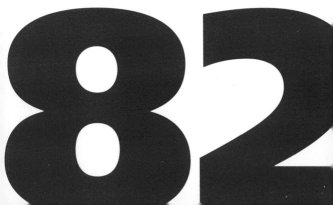

83 Get him to pay as much attention to the minors as the majors. According to a study by the Kinsey Institute, 98 per cent of women say they are as sensitive to having the labia minora, the delicate **inner lips** that surround the clitoris, stroked, as they are to direct clitoral stimulation.

84 Teach him how to multiply. A study from the Health Science Center at Brooklyn found that men can actually learn to climax and keep their erection through three to ten orgasms. The key lies in helping him raise his orgasmic threshold by constantly stimulating him until he's a heartbeat away from ejaculating, then stopping and resting before stimulating him again. The results should be **explosive**.

Get your **tongue** pierced. Apparently the stud is perfectly positioned to give extra friction on the most sensitive genital bits for men and women. Of course, you could try and create the same effect by slightly air-drying your tongue and sticking a frozen pea to it.

Masturbate in front of each other and find

out what really turns you on. 86

Make the **missionary** position work for you.
Start by changing the angle of his
dangle so that his penis pushes

87

up against the front wall of your vagina
and tickles your G-spot. This can be done by
slipping a small pillow under your hips or
having your lover place his hands underneath
your hips and lifting your whole pelvic area.

Show yourself. Men like to see naked women, which is why newspapers with topless models continue to flourish (although he STILL says he buys them for their thought-provoking articles). According to the US National Health and Social Life Survey, 50 per cent of men aged 18–44 find watching their partners undress 'very appealing'. Only vaginal intercourse ranked higher.

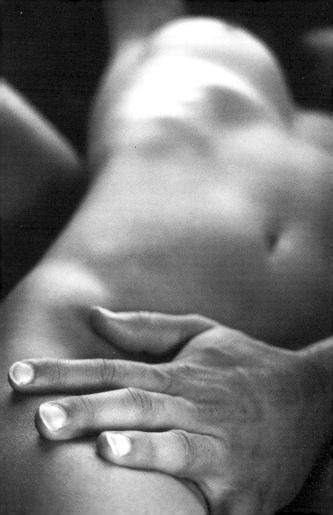

Plan a **romantic rendezvous** in October. This month sees the annual peak of testosterone in men, which explains why July (nine months later) is the busiest season for obstetricians.

Condoms don't have to interrupt your fun if you make putting them on a part of foreplay. Hold one very gently in your mouth, with the opening facing out. Then, using your tongue to help, gently roll it down your lover's penis with your lips (covering your lips with your teeth will prevent tears to the latex).

91

Access your **sexual chi** (energy) by practising the following ancient Indian breathing technique: block off your left nostril for 15 minutes (if you don't want to use your finger, a piece of cotton wool will do). This should redirect your airflow and ventilate the left side of your brain, which supposedly controls sexual arousal and creativity.

Have him try **The Venus** next time he gives you some oral stimulation. Ask him to alternate between lightly nibbling your clitoris, and flicking his tongue rapidly back and forth over the area. The result is a peel-you-off-the-ceiling kind of orgasm.

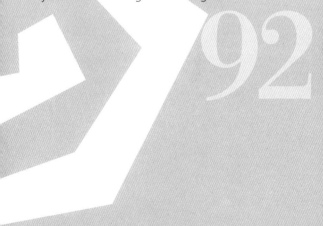

92

93 Make him climax faster than you can say, **'Fellatio'**. While sucking his penis, squeeze your thumb and index finger in an up-and-down motion along the ridge on the underside of the penile shaft. Then, using the same two fingers, squeeze under the sac of his balls, with each finger manipulating a ball in the same up-and-down motion (imagine you're milking a cow). You'll produce an orgasm with the intensity of two in a row.

94

Vibrational **energy** followers believe that the electromagnetic waves, naturally emitted by the earth, influence our body's rhythms. So if you're mentally and physically balanced, a magnet under your mattress will energize your orgasms.

Don't skip sex because you've got a headache or are suffering from PMS. Research from the Institute for the Advanced Study of Human Sexuality in San Francisco has found that a female orgasm is a **powerful painkiller** (thanks to the release of endorphins).

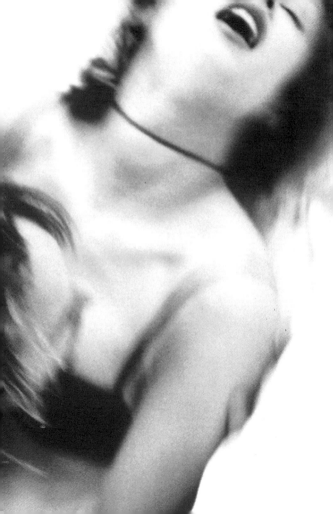

96 An easy way to help him last longer is to layer

his erection with **two** ultra-thin condoms. 96

Use birth control. It's impossible to relax and enjoy sex if you're worrying about getting pregnant, or contracting a sexually transmitted disease.

97

The sequence of touch can have an even more powerful **erotic effect** than the way you touch. Generally, it's most pleasurable to start by caressing the least sensitive or thicker-skinned places on your lover's body (such as the hips, buttocks, upper arms and shoulders), before working toward the more sensitive or thinner-skinned bits (such as the wrist, neck, inner thighs, lower spine, ears and temples).

98

99

Make up a sexual **fantasy together** – then put one of you in charge of 'producing' it. He or she must set the scene, gathering together props and arranging a 'preview' date.

100 Keep your diet bland. **What you eat** and drink hours before lovemaking strongly affects the way you both taste. Alcohol, garlic, saturated fats (like red meat), soy sauce and hot food give your secretions a bitter tang, while less spicy food produces a more neutral flavour. Sugar, on the other hand, will leave a sweet memory on the tongue.

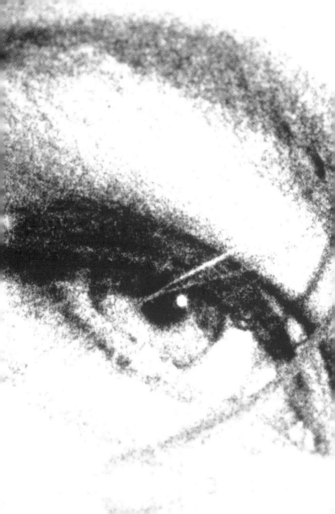

Teach him how to **blow you** with this simple move: during oral sex, ask him to place his lips so that they totally surround your clitoris. Then he should blow gently as though he were playing a trumpet. If he needs to take a breath, he should do so through his mouth. This way, he inhales and exhales on your clitoris, pushing it to climax after gorgeous climax.

101

102

To give your lovemaking a **sexy glow**, try blue light bulbs. They make the skin seem smoother, more touchable and radiant. Purple light, incidentally, magnifies sexual organs, making them appear larger than life. But skip red light. It makes you feel irritated and angry, as well as look artificial.

103 **Giftwrap** his penis in aluminium, but don't cook it. Instead, place your mouth over it, lightly touch your teeth to the foil and hum. It's a promise – he'll vibrate.

Share a **'melting hug'**. Hold each other very close for a long time. Nestle against one another's chests and wrap your arms gently around each other. Allow your thighs and bellies to meet. Let your bodies relax. Melt into each other's embrace. Let your own breathing harmonize with your partner's. After 30 minutes, you will feel a warm rush starting from the centre of your bodies and spreading outwards, before you both dissolve in an ecstatic mind-body-soul orgasm. **104**

Get

really

dirty and

then take a

shower together

in the dark. The

pulsating pressure of

the water is an effective

vibrator stand-in for both men

and women. But check the water

temperature first. **105**

Give each other head-to-toe **butterfly kisses**. Fluttering your eyelashes, roam each other's entire body, paying special attention to erogenous zones you've never considered before – the backs of the knees, the sensitive skin on either side of the Achilles tendon, the armpits and the jaw line.

107

Colour therapists recommend slipping into anything **red** to incite passion. But avoid lavender or green, as these shades will send you straight to sleep.

A man's penis is actually most sensitive immediately **AFTER** ejaculation. If you want to rev him up for another round, wait for five minutes after he's ejaculated, and then lightly caress the head of his penis with your tongue.

108

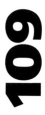

109

Skip commercial **lubricants**. They are often too sticky, and end up numbing all the luscious sensations by reducing friction. Instead, use your own saliva to moisten things – it's sexier and you always have a ready supply.

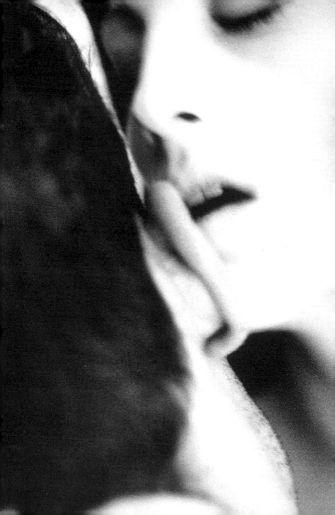

Unless you've been lost at sea for six months, **don't wash** before sex. You soap away your own natural, sexy scent. The French call the body's odour *la cassolette* (slang for perfume box), and view it as a huge turn-on for both men and women.

110